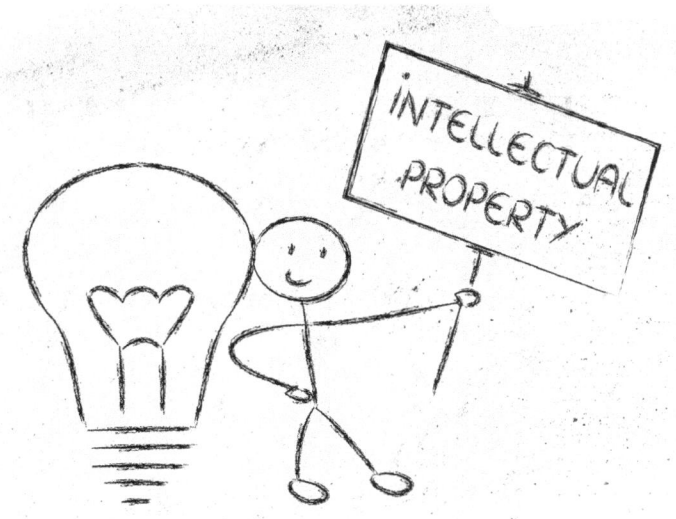

1

Table of Contents

Introduction

Most cooking enthusiasts and culinary aficionados will find that the majority of cook books focus on the mainline types of cooking methods. These cooking books contain recipes that the reader will cook using the normal methods that include frying, roasting and baking. However, this eBook covers one unique method the mainstream recipe and cooking books overlook. Crock pots, or slow cooking pots, are often overlooked since not many recipe and cooking books cover simmering methods of cooking.

How unique is the eBook?

While most cook book cover various recipes that use different cooking techniques, this eBook offers 50 recipes that rely on Crock Pot-based cooking techniques. Crock pots offer distinct advantages over other cooking methods. First, simmering preserves most of the nutrient value lost through frying and boiling. Additionally, this cooking method allows flavors to permeate through the food evenly.

The eBook offers advice on Crock pot cooking as well as various recipes that work best with this unique cooking method. Additionally, it advises the reader on the best methods as well as providing nutritional information that could benefit health-conscious readers. Foodies with weight management ambitions could also benefit since simmering does not use as much fat and oil as baking and frying.

Many cook books available today offer recipes for various foods that readers can prepare through different methods. Such books offer wide variety leaving little room for additional information that could benefit readers. One example of such is nutritional information, which the eBook offers in addition to the actual recipes. Such information makes the cook book a good resource for the modern health conscious reader or foodie.

- **Large variety of recipes, both conventional and unique**

Although Crock pot cooking can be used for a variety of foods ranging from breakfast to main dishes. The eBook will also teach the average reader to make BBQ-based dishes, various Mexican slow cook dishes, healthy slow cook dish options, Crock pot stews and soups, as well as main dishes. The eBook will make a good kitchen companion for the avid reader who is also eager to explore alternative methods of cooking. This important resource complements the current trend that seeks to change the unhealthy fixation on deep fried, bakes and processed pre-cooked foods. Reading this eBook should enable the average cook complement their skills set while increasing the healthy factor in their kitchen.

Creamy dip Artichoke and Parmesan

Ready in 2 hours.
8 portions
2 Points

INGREDIENTS

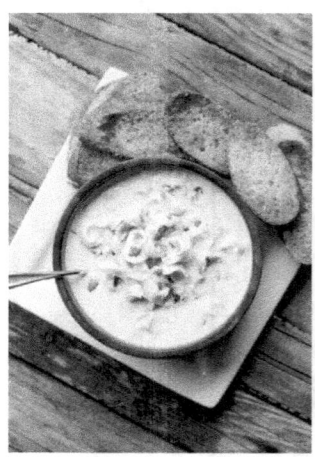

- 2 drained and chopped artichoke hearts boxes
- 2 cups shredded mozzarella cheese
- 1 1/2 cup grated Parmesan cheese
- 1 1/2 cup mayonnaise
- 1/2 cup finely chopped onion
- 1/2 c. with dried oregano
- 1/4 c. tea garlic powder
- 4 pitas
- pre-cut mixed vegetables

PREPARATION
1. Combine artichoke hearts, cheese, mayonnaise, onion, and garlic powder and in a slow cooker and mix well.
2. Cover and cook on low for 2 hours.
3. During cooking, cut pita bread into triangles. Arrange vegetables and the pita bread and on a plate and serve with the warm dip.

Nutrition information
Calories: 60.9
Fats: 4.3g
Carbohydrates: 3.1g
Proteins: 2.3g

Rice Pudding Recipe

Ready in 1h 35 min.
8 Portions
4 Points

INGREDIENTS
- 2 cups milk
- 1 can (370 ml) evaporated milk
- 1/2 c. cinnamon tea
- 5 c. table sugar
- 2/3 cup raisins
- 1 1/2 cup Uncle Ben's rice already cooked
- 3 eggs, beaten

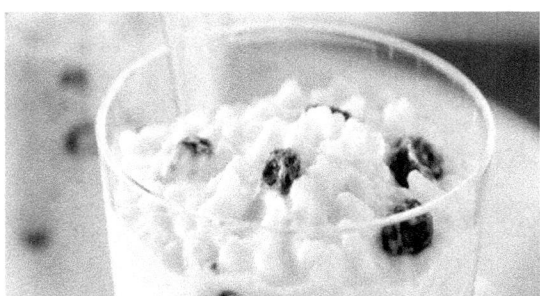

PREPARATION
1. Coat the crock pot with a thin layer of cooking spray. Place the milk in the crock pot and cinnamon, raisins and sugar. Put it under high temperature.Cover and cook 1:30, stirring occasionally.
2. When everything is hot and it is simmering, stir well and add the beaten eggs, stirring constantly with a whisk.
3. Within minutes, the liquid will be thickened cream. Add the rice already cooked and remove the container from slow cooker.
4. Cool and serve with a touch of maple syrup

Nutrition information
Calories: 142
Fats: 2.1g
Carbohydrates: 27g
Proteins: 4.2g

Macaroni and cheese

Ready in 6 h 10 min.
6 Servings
8 Points

INGREDIENTS
- 1 cup uncooked macaroni
- 4 cups Cheddar cheese, grated, divided
- 1 can (370 ml) evaporated milk
- 1 ½ cup milk
- 2 eggs
- 1 c. teaspoon salt
- 1/2 c. pepper tea

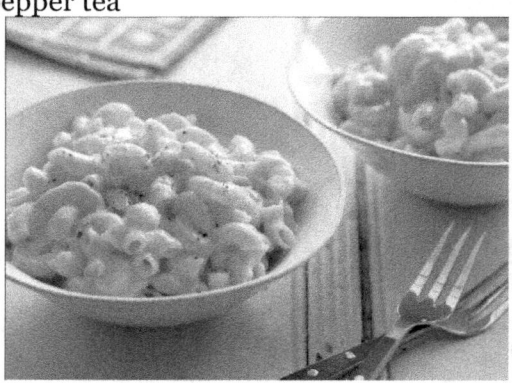

PREPARATION
1. Grease the inside of the bowl of the slow cooker with cooking spray and spray.
2. In a large bowl, beat eggs, evaporated milk, and milk. Add uncooked macaroni and 3 cups shredded cheese. Transfer the bowl in the slow cooker. Sprinkle remaining grated cheese on top.
3. Cook on low heat for 5-6 hours.
4. Do not lift the lid during cooking.

Nutrition information
Calories: 310
Fats: 9g
Carbohydrates: 44g
Proteins: 13g

Chickpea Ratatouille

Prep Time: 10 minutes. Cook Time: 4hours. 20 minutes
Servings: 6
7 Points

INGREDIENTS
- 1 c. in vegetable oil
- 1 chopped onion
- 2 garlic cloves, finely chopped
- 1 large eggplant, diced
- 2 c. dried basil tea
- 1 c. with dried oregano
- 1/2 c. Salt tea
- 1/2 c. black pepper tea mill
- 1 can whole tomatoes (28 oz.)
- 2 peppers, cut into 1-inch
- 2 zucchini,
- 1/3 cup tomato paste
- 1 chickpeas, drained and rinsed
- 2 cups cooked chickpeas house
- 1/4 cup basil or chopped fresh parsley

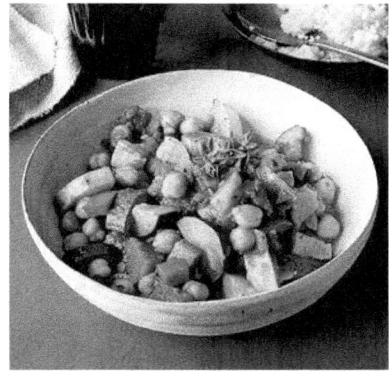

PREPARATION
1. In a large skillet, heat oil over medium heat. Add onion, garlic, eggplant, dried basil, oregano, salt and pepper and cook, stirring occasionally, for about 10 minutes or until onion is softened. Put the mixture in slow cooker.
2. Add tomatoes, breaking up with a wooden spoon and peppers, zucchini, tomato paste and chickpeas. Cover and cook on low for 4 hours. (You can prepare ratatouille until this stage, let cool completely and place in airtight containers. It will keep for up to 3 days in the refrigerator or freezer up to 1 month.)
3. Add the basil and mix.

Nutrition information
Calories: 268
Fats: 19g
Carbohydrates: 11g
Proteins: 13g

Spaghetti sauce

Prep Time: 10 minutes. Cook Time: 3hours. 20 minutes
Servings: 32
5 Points

INGREDIENTS
- 4 chopped onions
- 4 cloves garlic, minced
- 1 green pepper, chopped
- 1/2 cup vegetable oil
- 16 cups chopped tomato
- 2 c. tablespoons dried oregano
- 2 c. dried basil soup
- 1/4 cup chopped fresh parsley
- 1/4 cup sugar
- 2 c. tablespoon salt
- 3/4 c. pepper tea
- 1 can tomato paste

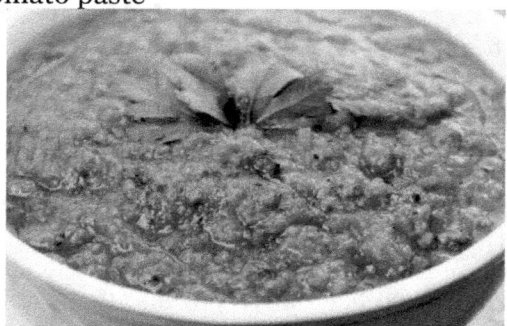

PREPARATION
1. In a skillet, fry the onion, garlic and peppers in the vegetable oil for 5 minutes. Transfer to a slow cooker.
2. Add tomatoes, oregano, basil, parsley, sugar, salt and pepper. Cook 2-3 hours on low power. Stir frequently.
3. Allow the sauce cooling. Spoon into freezer containers to freeze
4. At the time of consuming the sauce, heat by adding 156 ml of tomato paste.

Nutrition information
Calories: 202
Fats: 1.5g
Carbohydrates: 40g
Proteins: 7g

House marinara sauce

Prep Time: 20 minutes. Cook Time: 8 hours.
Servings: 12
1 Point

INGREDIENTS
- 1/4 cup canola oil
- 1 medium onion, chopped
- 10 oz. crushed tomatoes
- 1 cup tomato sauce
- 3 oz. tomato paste
- 2 ½ c. tablespoon garlic powder
- 2 tablespoons dried oregano
- 2 c. dried basil soup
- 2 tablespoons sugar
- 2 teaspoon salt
- 2 teaspoon ground black pepper

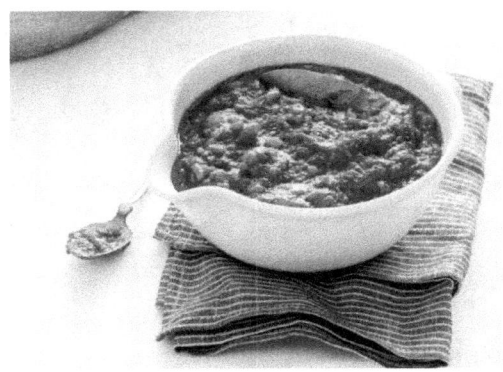

PREPARATIONS
1. Heat canola oil in a skillet over medium heat and fry the onion in oil until soft.
2. In the bowl of a slow cooker, combine the cooked onions with remaining ingredients.
3. Cover and cook on low heat for 8 hours.

Nutrition information
Calories: 40
Fats: 1g
Carbohydrates: 8g
Proteins: 1g

Creamy spinach

Ready in 5 h 20 min.
8 servings
7 Points

INGREDIENTS

- 2 packages (300 g each) of frozen spinach thawed and squeezed to drain
- 2 cups cottage cheese
- 1/2 cup butter into cubes
- 3 eggs, beaten
- 1 1/2 cup yellow cheese
- 1/4 cup all-purpose flour
- 1 c. teaspoon salt

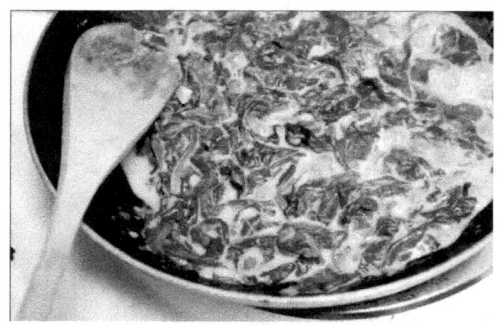

PREPARATION

1. Grease the bowl of a slow cooker. In a large bowl, put together the spinach, cottage cheese, butter, yellow cheese, eggs, flour and salt.
2. Mix well. Transfer to slow cooker.
3. Cook on High heat for 1 hour, then reduce to low heat and cook for 4-5 hours.

Nutrition information
Calories: 240
Fats: 19g
Carbohydrates: 12g
Proteins: 10g

Macaroni and cheese with broccoli

Ready in 4 h 10 min.
10 servings
9 Points

INGREDIENTS
- Vegetable oil spray
- 7 oz. of uncooked macaroni
- 1 c. tablespoons vegetable oil
- 4 cups Cheddar cheese, grated
- 2 sticks (370 ml) evaporated milk (Carnation style)
- 3 cups milk
- 1 bag frozen broccoli, thawed
- Salt and pepper to taste

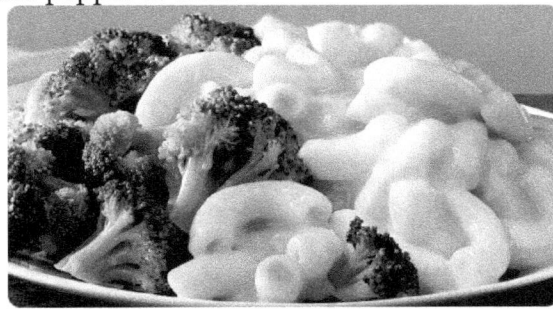

PREPARATION
1. Smear oil inside the bowl of the slow cooker with spray oil. Add macaroni and 1 c. tablespoons oil and mix to cover oil macaroni.
2. Add Cheddar cheese, evaporated milk, milk, broccoli, salt and pepper; mix.
3. Cover and cook on low heat (LOW) for 4-5 hours, stirring occasionally to prevent it from sticking.
4. Spread the slices of zucchini and onions into the bowl of slow cooker.
5. Add the cubes of butter and cheese cubes.
6. Cook on low heat (LOW) about 1 hour. Do not mix.

Nutrition information
Calories: 190
Fats: 5g
Carbohydrates: 44g
Proteins: 9g

Ginger-Chicken Noodle Soup

Ready in 4 hours 15 minutes.
4 servings
4 Points
INREDIENTS

- 2 pounds skinless, boneless chicken thighs
- 4 medium carrots, roughly shredded
- 4 tablespoons dry sherry
- 2 tablespoon soy sauce
- 2 tablespoon rice vinegar
- 2 teaspoon grated fresh ginger
- 1/2 teaspoon black pepper (ground)
- 5-15 - ounce can chicken broth
- 2 cups of water
- 18 - Ounce package frozen pea pods

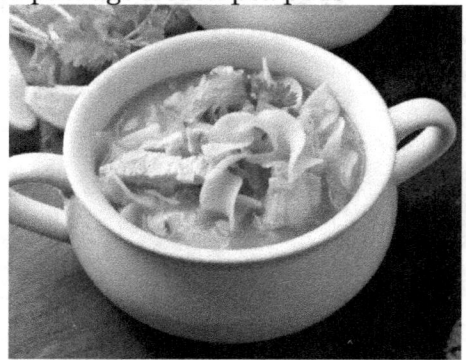

PREPARATION

1. Combine chicken, carrots, sherry, vinegar, ginger, and pepper.
2. Stir in chicken broth and the water.
3. Cover and cook on high-heat setting for 4 hours.
4. Stir in noodles and pea pods.
5. Cover and cook for 10 to 15 minutes more or until noodles are tender.
6. Serve with additional soy sauce.

Nutrition information
Calories: 143
Fats: 3g
Carbohydrates: 12g
Proteins: 17g

Pulled pork

Ready in 9 h 15 min.
6 servings
11 Points

INGREDIENTS
- 2 lb. roast pork shoulder
- Salt
- pepper
- 1/2 cup ketchup
- 1/2 cup brown sugar
- 1/3 cup red wine vinegar

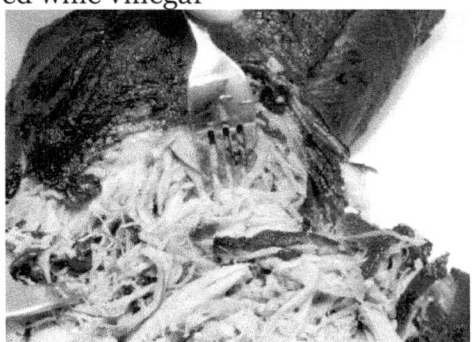

PREPARATION
1. Preheat the slow cooker to low power for 15 minutes
2. Add salt and pepper to the roast pork and place in slow cooker. Mix the ketchup, brown sugar and vinegar in a bowl. Pour meat in the over.
3. Cook for 8 hours on low heat.
4. Transfer roast to a platter and cut into 3 or four large pieces.
5. Shred meat with two forks and put in the slow cooker for 1 hour.

Nutrition information
Calories: 417
Fats: 11g
Carbohydrates: 47g
Proteins: 33g

Roast Beef

Ready in 4h 15 min.
8 servings
32 Points

Ingredients
- 2 lb. roast beef
- 1 c. tablespoon salt
- 1 c. tablespoons ground black pepper
- 2 c. in dried parsley tea
- 2 c. dried oregano tea
- 4 potatoes, chopped
- 2 cups baby carrots
- 1 tomato, chopped
- 1/2 yellow onion, chopped
- 1 can tomato sauce
- 1/2 cup water

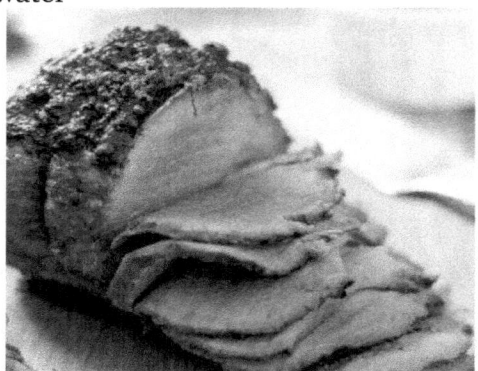

PREPARATION
1. Sprinkle salt roast, pepper, parsley and oregano on roast beef. Place in slow cooker and add the potato chunks, carrots, tomatoes and onion.
2. Pour the tomato sauce and water on top.
3. Cover and cook on high (HIGH) for 4 hours.

Nutrition information
Calories: 1303
Fats: 45g
Carbohydrates: 0g
Proteins: 224g

Quinoa porridge, vanilla and raisins

Prep time 5 min. Cooking time; 8h.
4 servings
7 Points

INGREDIENTS
- 1/2 cup quinoa
- 2 1/2 cups of soy milk with vanilla
- 1/4 cup of grapes (or cranberries)
- 1/2 cup of unsweetened applesauce
- 1/2 teaspoon of vanilla extract
- Nuts or seeds to be used (OPTIONAL)
- Cinnamon to serve (optional)

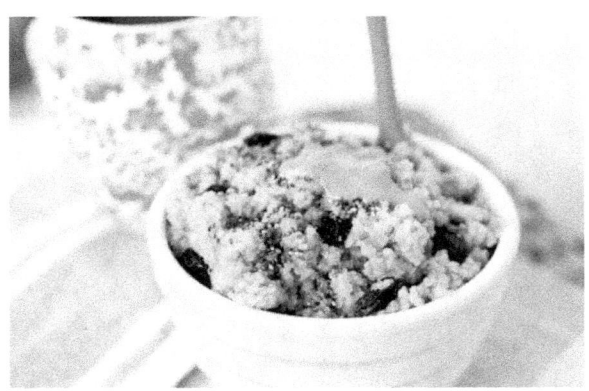

PREPARATION
   Just drop everything in the Slow Cooker and cook "low" for about
   6-8 hours.

Nutrition information
Calories: 265.5
Fats: 5.8g
Carbohydrates: 45.7g
Proteins: 8.4g

Pumpkin porridge

Prep time 5 min. Cooking time; 8h.
4 servings
6 Points

INGREDIENTS
- 2.5 Cups of almond milk
- 1 Cup Pumpkin Puree
- 1 Cup of Crushed Oats
- 1 Cup of Agave syrup or liquid honey
- 1 spoon Spices mixed Café Gingerbread
- broken pecans (for the service)

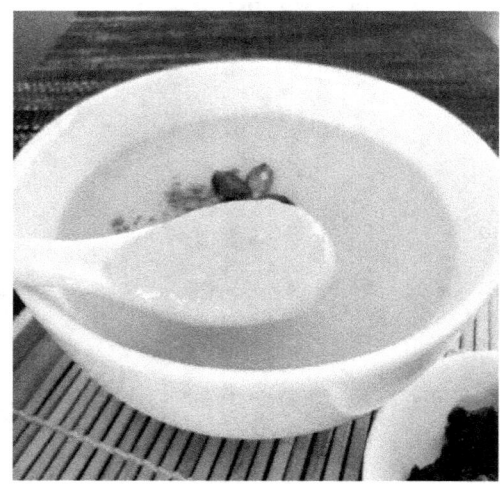

PREPARATION
1. Put all the ingredients (except the pecans) in the slow cooker, set the cooking for 8 hours the mildest temperature (low).
2. Once cooked, divide into bowls, drizzle with honey or agave syrup, optionally adding chopped pecans and serve warm or cold.

Nutrition information
Calories: 211
Fats: 3g
Carbohydrates: 44g
Proteins: 4g

Prep time 5 min. Cooking time; 3h.
4 servings
5 Points

INGREDIENTS
- 2 cups warm water
- 1 package of active dry yeast
- 1 c table sugar
- 3 1/2 cups plain flour
- 1/2 tsp. teaspoon salt
- 2 tablespoons oil table
- Almond Milk

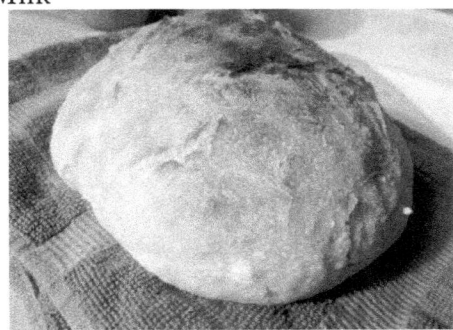

PREPARATION
1. Preheat slow cooker to HIGH with the lid closed. Dissolve yeast in 1/2 cup warm water with sugar and put in a warm place.
2. Put the flour in a large bowl and sprinkle with salt. Make a well in center. When yeast is bubbling: put the rest of the water and the add oil into the flour. Stir with your fingers until all the flour is absorbed. Grease a pan and put the bread crumbs. Top with almond milk.
3. Cover with a plate and let stand for 5 minutes in a warm place. Place on a trivet (support) in the slow cooker, cover and cook for 2-3 hours.

Nutrition information
Calories: 163
Fats: 3.9g
Carbohydrates: 27.8g
Proteins: 6.4g

Beef stew

Ready in 6 h 35 minutes.
6 portions
5 Points

INGREDIENTS
- 2 c. tab in vegetable oil
- 2 lb. stewing beef cubes
- 2 onions, chopped
- 2 c. tab in chili
- 1 c. sea salt
- 1 c. black pepper
- 4 carrots, cut into 1-inch (2.5 cm)
- 4 stalks celery, cut into 1-inch (2.5 cm)
- 1 c. to tab cider vinegar
- 1 c. tab in liquid honey
- 1 3/4 cup beef broth
- 1/3 cup flour
- 1/2 cup water
- 1 1/2 cups frozen corn kernels
- 1 1/2 cup frozen lima beans

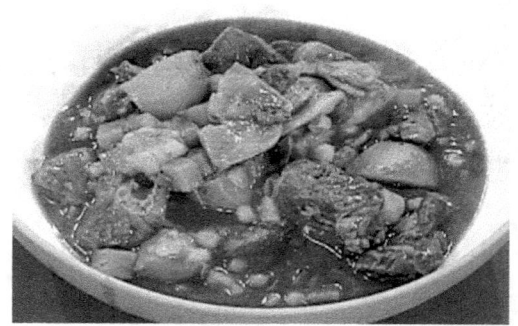

PREPARATION

1. In a large skillet, heat half the oil over medium-high heat. Add the cubes of beef, in batches, and brown them. Put the beef in the slow cooker.
2. Degrease the pan. Heat the remaining oil over medium heat. Add onions, chili powder, salt and pepper and cook, stirring occasionally, for about 4 minutes or until onions are softened.
3. Put the mixture in slow cooker. Add carrots, celery, apple cider vinegar and honey.
4. In the skillet, add 1 cup (250 ml) of broth and bring to boil, scraping the bottom to loosen particles. Pour this liquid in the slow cooker, then add the remaining broth.
5. Cover and cook on low for 6 to 8 hours. Degrease the preparation.
6. In a small bowl, mix the flour and water, pour into the slow cooker and stir well. Cover and cook on high heat until sauce is thickened. (You can prepare the stew until this stage, let it cool completely and place in airtight containers. It will keep up to 3 days in the refrigerator or freezer up to 1 month.)
7. Add corn and lima beans and mix. Cover and cook until the stew is steaming.

Nutrition information
Calories: 207
Fats: 6g
Carbohydrates: 22g
Proteins: 17g

Casserole of pork chops and rice

Ready in 1 hour 12 minutes.
4 portions
12 Points

INGREDIENTS
- 4 pork loin chops with the bone
- 1/2tsp. salt
- 1/2tsp. ground black pepper
- 1 c. to tab vegetable oil
- 3/4 cup of sausage
- 1 sliced onion
- 1 red pepper
- 1tsp. dried thyme
- 3/4 cup long-grain rice
- 1 1/2 cups chicken broth
- 2 green onions, sliced

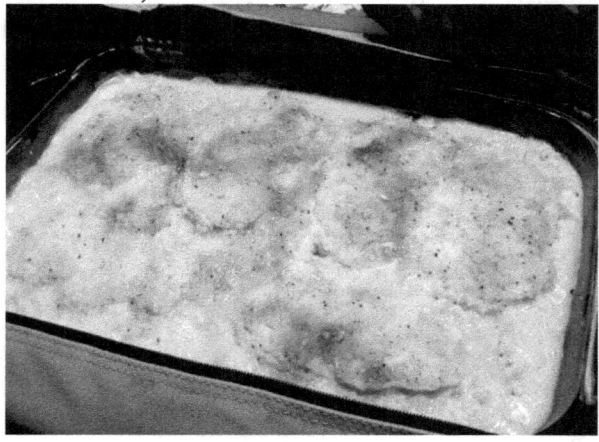

PREPARATION

1. Sprinkle pork chops with half the salt and pepper. In a large metal pot, heat oil over medium-high heat. Add the pork chops and cook for about 4 minutes or until browned (return in mid-cooking). Remove chops from the pan and reserve.

2. Degrease the casserole. Add the sausage, onion, red pepper, thyme and remaining salt and pepper and cook over medium heat, stirring occasionally until onion is softened. Pour the rice and cook while stirring for 1 minute to coat well. Pour the chicken broth. Arrange the reserved pork chops over rice and bring to a boil.

3. Cover the casserole and bake in preheated 375 ° F (190 ° C) for about 1 hour or until pork is tender. (You can prepare the pan in advance, let it cool in the pan uncovered, and then cover. It will keep for up to 2 days in the refrigerator. To freeze, wrap the pan and cover with foil, then slip it into a large Ziploc freezer bag. The pan will keep up to 2 months in the freezer. to reheat, thaw in the refrigerator the night before and bake at 325 ° F / 160 ° C for about 40 minutes.)

4. Before serving, sprinkle with green onions.

Nutrition information
Calories: 455.7
Fats: 12.9g
Carbohydrates: 53.2g
Proteins: 30g

Cassoulet with chicken and pork

Ready in 7 h 30 min.
8 servings
8 Points

INGREDIENTS

- 3 c. tab in vegetable oil
- 2 lb.chicken thighs
- 1 roasted boneless pork shoulder
- 1 chopped onion
- 2 cloves garlic, crushed
- 1 diced tomatoes, drained
- 1 1/2 cup chicken broth salt reduced
- 1 cup dry white wine
- 1 c. tab in tomato paste
- 2 sprigs of fresh thyme
- 1 bay leaf
- 1/2 lb. cooked pork sausages1 cup bread crumbs
- 19 oz. of white beans
- 1/2 c. with fresh thyme tea, chopped
- 1/2 c. Salt tea
- 1/2 c. black pepper

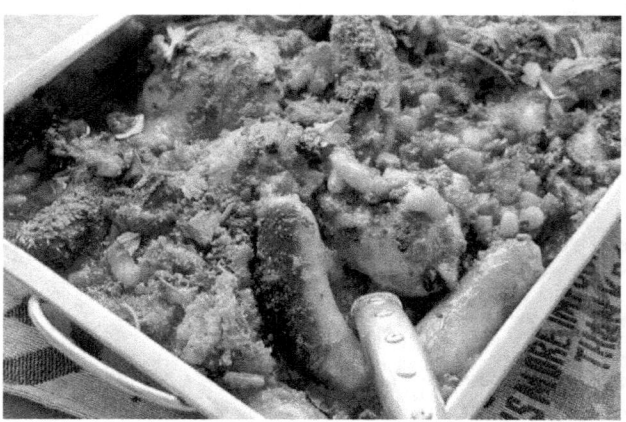

PREPARATION
1. In a large skillet, heat oil over medium-high heat. Add the chicken thighs high and cubes of pork, in batches, and brown them. Place chicken and pork in slow cooker. Add onion, garlic, tomatoes, broth, wine, tomato paste, thyme sprigs and bay leaf.
2. Cover and cook on low for 7 hours.
3. Add sausage, 3/4 cup (180 ml) bread crumbs, white beans, chopped thyme, salt and pepper and mix. Cover and continue cooking at high intensity for 15 minutes. Remove thyme sprigs and bay leaf. (You can prepare cassoulet in advance, let it cool completely and place in airtight containers. It will keep up to 3 days in the refrigerator or freezer up to 1 month.)
4. Just before serving, sprinkle each serving with 1/2 c. in tab (7 mL) of the remaining crumbs.

Nutrition information
Calories: 350
Fats: 11g
Carbohydrates: 30g
Proteins: 21g

Beef braised in beer

Ready in 2 h 30 minutes.
4 servings
6 Points

INGREDIENTS
- 2 lb. approximately beef chuck roast
- Salt and freshly ground pepper
- 3 tbsp. Vegetable oil
- 2 tbsp. Of butter
- 3 cups sliced leeks
- 3 oz. of minced smoked bacon
- 2 chopped cloves of garlic
- 1 punnet of mushrooms cut into four
- 1 cup of lager
- 2 bay leaves
- ½ cup Dijon mustard
- ½ cup chopped parsley

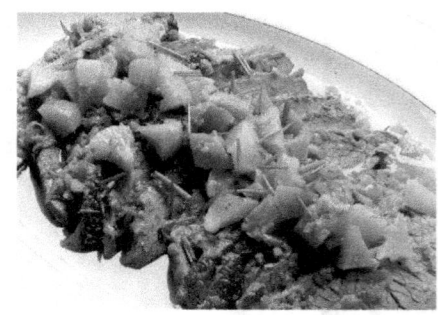

PREPARATION
1. Preheat oven to 180 C (350 F) .Heat the pot at the maximum temperature in the oven, add oil and butter. Fry the beef roast on both sides.
2. Remove from heat, add leeks, bacon, mushrooms and garlic. Fry for 2 minutes. Pour beer.
3. Bake for 2 hours. At the end of cooking, add the mustard and chopped parsley.
4. Return to oven and cook for 20 minutes.
5. Can be cooked in a slow cooker for 8 hours at medium temperature.

Nutrition information
Calories: 240
Fats: 6g
Carbohydrates: 23g
Proteins: 23g

Cigar cabbage

Ready in 6h 15 minutes
6 portions
4 Points

INGREDIENTS
- 1 1/2 lb. lean minced meat. mixture of beef, pork and veal
- 1 c. celery
- salt
- 1 c. dried oregano
- 1 c. dried basil tea
- 1/2 small finely grated carrot
- 1 onion, finely chopped
- 1/2 cup water or beef broth
- 1/4 cup uncooked white or brown rice
- 1/2 c. garlic powder
- 2 yolks, lightly beaten eggs
- Salt and pepper to taste
- Sauce :
- 26 oz. tomatoes
- Salt and pepper to taste
- 1 c. tablespoons brown sugar
- 1 c. tablespoon lemon juice
- 2 bay leaves
- 8-12 large cabbage leaves

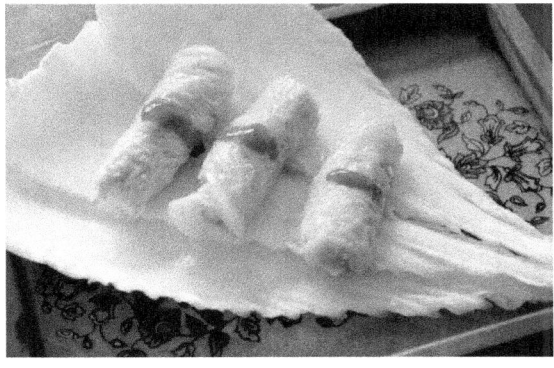

PREPARATION
1. Boil cabbage leaves in salted water for 5 minutes. Meanwhile, mix all the stuffing ingredients.
2. Pat the cabbage leaves, then stuff the meat. Roll up for cigars and put a toothpick to hold together. Place the cigar in slow cooker.
3. In a large bowl, combine all sauce ingredients. Pour the sauce over the cigars.
4. Close the lid of the slow cooker and simmer for 6 hours at low temperature or 3 hours at high temperature.

Nutrition information
Calories: 161.2
Fats: 10.1g
Carbohydrates: 9g
Proteins: 8.9g

American beef Stew

Ready in 12h 15 min.
4 portions
9 Points

INGREDIENTS
- 2 lb. beef cubes
- 1/4 cup all-purpose flour
- 1 c. paprika
- 1/2 c. pepper tea
- 1 bay leaf
- 1 garlic clove
- 3 diced potatoes
- 1 foot sliced celery
- 2 onions, chopped
- 1 c. Tea soy sauce
- 375ml beef stock

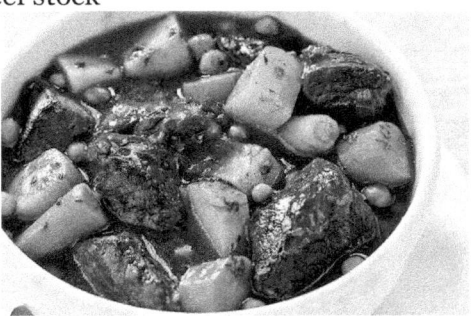

PREPARATION
1. In a bowl, mix together flour, paprika and pepper.
2. Coat beef cubes.
3. Place the beef in a slow cooker. Add the rest of the ingredients and mix well.
4. Cook at for 4-6 hours at high temperature for or low temperature of 10 to 12 hours.

Nutrition information
Calories: 350
Fats: 12g
Carbohydrates: 28g
Proteins: 33g

Braised beef with ginger

Ready in 8 h 30 minutes.
6 servings
5 Points

INGREDIENTS

- 6 lb. roast beef
- 1/2 c. ground black pepper
- 2 tbsp. table vegetable oil
- 1 onion,
- 5 cloves garlic
- 1 tbsp. fresh ginger, finely chopped
- 1/2 cup hoisin sauce
- 1/2 cup beef broth
- 1/4 cup packed brown sugar
- 1/4 cup soy sauce
- 1/2 cup water
- 2 tbsp. table flour
- 2 shallots

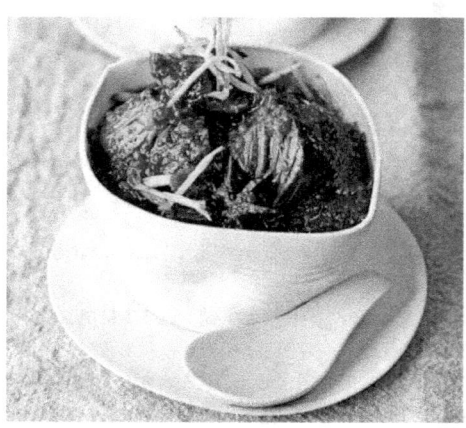

PREPARATION
1. Sprinkle roast beef with pepper. In a skillet, heat oil over medium-high heat.
2. Add roast and brown on all sides. Put the roast beef in slow cooker.
   Degrease the pan. Add onion, garlic and ginger and cook over medium heat, stirring occasionally, for 2 minutes or until onion is softened.
3. Add hoisin sauce, beef broth, brown sugar, soy sauce and half of the water and stir, scraping the bottom of the pan to loosen the particles. Pour into slow cooker. Cover and cook on low heat for 8 to 10 hours.
4. Place roast on a cutting board and cover with foil loosely. Let stand for 10 minutes. Cut the roast beef into thin slices and place in a serving dish. Cover to keep warm.
5. Meanwhile, scouring the cooking liquid. In a bowl, mix flour and remaining water. Pour flour in slow cooker and mix. Cover and cook on high for 15 minutes or until sauce is thickened (stir once during cooking). Coat the sliced roast reserved sauce. Garnish with green onions.

Nutrition information
Calories: 207
Fats: 8g
Carbohydrates: 10.3g
Proteins: 22.9g

Cheese sauce and meat.

Ready in 2h.
8 servings
11 Points

INGREDIENTS

- 1 lb. lean ground beef
- 1 onion, chopped
- 1 tbsp. Butter
- 1 tbsp. Chili powder
- 1 tsp. Ground cumin
- 1/2 cup of lager
- 1 lb. Velveeta cheese, cubed
- 14 oz. diced tomatoes
- 1 pepper
- Salt

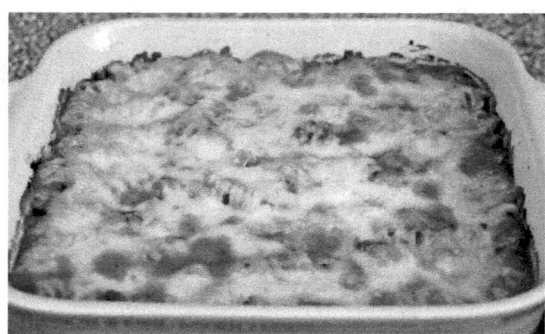

PREPARATION

1. Brown the meat and onion in butter in a large nonstick skillet over medium-high heat.
2. Add spices and cook for 2 minutes. Add salt and pepper. Deglaze with the beer.
3. Transfer to slow cooker.
4. Add remaining ingredients and mix. Cover and cook at low temperature (Low) for 2 hours.
5. Stir well before serving, directly into the slow cooker. Serve with corn chips.

Nutrition information
Calories: 364
Fats: 30g
Carbohydrates: 20g
Proteins: 11g

Ready in 6h 20 minutes.
5 servings
8 Points

INGREDIENTS
- 1 whole chicken
- 4 potatoes cut into quarters
- 4 carrots, cut into 2-inch pieces
- 1 large onion, sliced
- 1 bag barbecue sauce
- 1 cup chicken broth
- Chicken with spices
- Vegetables spices
- Roasted garlic
- Peppers
- Salt

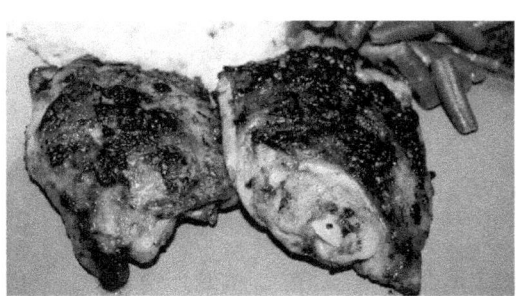

PREPARATION
1. Place onion in bottom of slow cooker and place the chicken on top.
2. Combine chicken broth, water and the bag of barbecue sauce and pour over the chicken (it should have about 1 inch in cash and half in bottom of slow cooker).
3. Put all the vegetables around chicken and add spices to taste. Cook on low heat for 6 hours without opening the slow cooker to keep in heat.
4. Serve with the reduced sauce of slow cooker or barbecue sauce trade.

Nutrition information
Calories: 320
Fats: 16g
Carbohydrates: 2.4g
Proteins: 40g

Pork with cider

Ready in 12h 35 min.
4 portions
7 Points

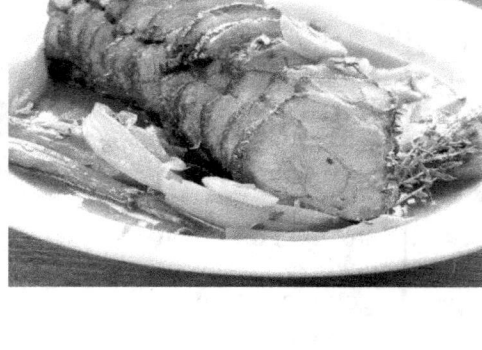

INGREDIENTS
- 2 lb. pork cubes
- 3 c. tablespoons all-purpose flour
- 1 c. Salt tea
- 1/4 c. thyme
- 1/4 c. pepper
- 6 sliced carrots
- 4 sliced potatoes
- 2 chopped onions
- 1 diced apple
- 2 cups apple cider or apple juice
- 1 c. tablespoons white vinegar
- 1/2 cup cold water

PREPARATION
1. Combine 3 tbsp. tablespoons (24 grams) of flour with salt, pepper and thyme and then cover with the meat.
2. Place vegetables and apples in the slow cooker.
3. Top with pork cubes
4. Mix apple cider and vinegar and pour over meat.
5. Cover and cook on low heat for 10 to 12 hours.
6. Cook in high temperature and mix the flour and water.
7. Pour and stir the stew liquid.
8. Cover and cook 15 minutes, or until sauce is thick.

Nutrition information
Calories: 281.4
Fats: 8.4g
Carbohydrates: 29.4g
Proteins: 22.7g

Spaghetti Sauce

Ready in 4 h 25 min.
12 portions
5 points

INGREDIENTS
- 3lb. g ground beef
- 1 cup mushrooms
- 4 cups frozen vegetables
- 1 1/2 tomatoes box
- 3 boxes of five ounces tomato paste
- 3 bay leaves
- 3/8 c. Tea paprika
- 3/8 c. with oregano
- 1/8 c. cayenne pepper tea
- 3/4 c. Tea garlic salt
- 3/4 c. Herb tea Provence
- 3 c. sugar or maple syrup table

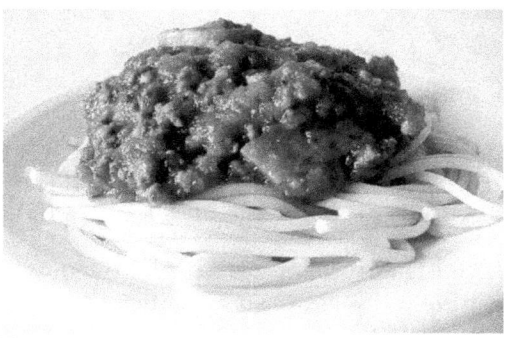

PREPARATION
1. Brown the meat and place in a slow cooker.
2. Add the remaining ingredients and cook for 4 hours at high temperature.

Nutrition information
Calories: 202
Fats: 1.5g
Carbohydrates: 40g
Proteins: 7g

Bread Dish Lost Cinnamon

Prep time 30 minutes. Cooking time 3hrs.
4 servings
2 Points

INGREDIENTS
- 6 cups bread cinnamon scrolls, cubed
- 7 large eggs
- 2 tablespoons of lemon juice
- ¼ cup sugar
- ¼ cup maple syrup
- 2 tbsp. in pure vanilla extract
- 1½ tea. with ground cinnamon
- ¼ tsp. with ground nutmeg
- 7/8 cup vegetable oil
- ¾ cup dates, chopped
- ¾ cup caramelized pecans,
- 2 tsp. teaspoon brown sugar
- 1 cup chopped pecans

PREPARATION
1. Spray the inside of your Crock-Pot with nonstick cooking spray.
2. Spread the bread cubes on a baking sheet. Let them brown in the oven at 275 ° F for 20 minutes or until they are lightly dried and cured. Transfer the bread cubes in your slow cooker.
3. During cooking cubes of bread in the oven, whisk eggs, sugar, maple syrup, vanilla, cinnamon and nutmeg in a mixing bowl
4. Pour the mixture over the bread and stir gently to ensure that all cubes are submerged. Sprinkle with dates and pecans (melt the butter and brown sugar and pecans coat of this mixture; bake until completely caramelized). Finish with the pieces of butter.
5. Cook over high heat for 3 to 4 hours. Garnish with powdered sugar and syrup. Enjoy your meal!

Nutrition information
Calories: 90
Fats: 2.5g
Carbohydrates: 14g
Proteins: 3g

Prep time 10 minutes. Cooking time, 6 hours.
6 Servings
16 Points

INGREDIENTS
- 1 package (28 ounces) of potatoes
- 1½ cup cheese (Mexican blend), grated
- 1 lb. country style sausage
- 12 large eggs
- 1 tablespoon lemon juice

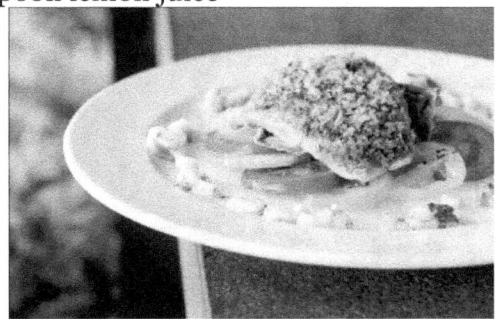

PREPARATION
1. Crumble the sausage meat and let it brown in a skillet.
2. Transfer to a bowl and use a paper towel to remove most of the fat.
3. Beat the eggs in a mixing bowl.
4. Spray the container of your Crock-Pot with nonstick cooking spray.
5. Place the ingredients in your slow cooker in the order of the list of ingredients.
6. Cook over low heat for 6 to 8 hours
7. Serve with salsa, salt and pepper to taste.

Nutrition information
Calories: 612
Fats: 40g
Carbohydrates: 37g
Proteins: 27g

Jook Oatmeal

Prep time, 10 min. Cooking time, 4 hrs.
4 servings
3 Points

INGREDIENTS
- 1 cup steel-cut oats
- 1-2 c. tablespoon sesame oil
- 2-3 cloves garlic, chopped
- 2 to 3 tbsp. chopped fresh ginger,
- 5-6 green onions
- 1 pinch of cayenne pepper (optional)
- 3 chicken bouillon cups
- 1 pea cup and frozen carrots Filling:
- White pepper
- Peanuts
- Roasted almonds
- Sesame oil

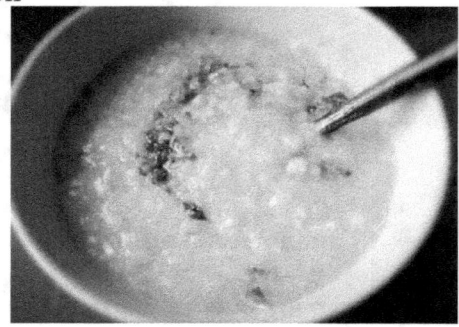

PREPARATION
1. Place all ingredients except green onion sections and frozen peas and carrots in your Crock-Pot. Mix.
2. Cook over low heat for 8-9 hours or on high heat for 3 to 4 hours.
3. About 1 hour before the end of cooking, add the frozen peas and carrots.
4. Garnish with green onion sections and any other ingredient of your choice.

Nutrition information
Calories: 138
Fats: 1.3g
Carbohydrates: 28g
Proteins: 1.3g

Ready in 3 h 30 min.
4 portions.
7 Points

INGREDIENTS

- 2 cans of canned tomato soup.
- 2 cups of boiling water (depending on desired consistency)
- 4 tablespoons of concentrated beef broth
- 1 tablespoon pepper
- 1 tablespoons sugar
- 1 pinch thyme
- 1 pinch basil
- 1 pinch of oregano
- 1 pinch spices Italian
- 1 lb. ground beef
- 1 chopped celery
- 1/2 onion, chopped
- 1 egg

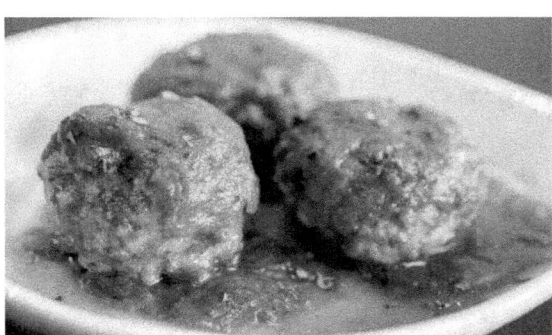

PREPARATION

1. Prepare the broth into slow cooker. Mix tomato soup, boiling water, concentrated beef broth, pepper and sugar. Add herbs and mix well.
2. Chop the meat grinder celery and onion. Mix with minced meat and egg. Roll balls in the desired size.
3. Put the meatballs into slow cooker and cover well the broth. Cook over high intensity 3 hours.

Nutrition information
Calories: 284
Fats: 13g
Carbohydrates: 12g
Proteins: 30g

Meat bread

Ready in 6h 15 minutes.
6 portions.
6 Points

INGREDIENTS
Meatloaf:
- 1 lb. extra lean ground beef
- 1/2 lb. extra lean ground pork
- 1/2 lb. extra lean ground veal
- 1/2 c. Tea onion powder
- 1/4 c. celery salt tea
- 2 eggs
- 1/2 cup tomato sauce
- 3/4 cup of breadcrumbs
- 1/2 c. ground savory
- 1/8 c. ground nutmeg
- Salt and pepper

Sauce:
- 7 oz. Diced tomatoes
- 5 oz. tomato sauce
- Salt and pepper

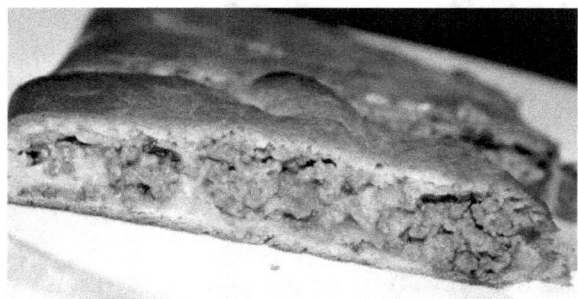

PREPARATION
1. Mix the first 11 ingredients with hands until well blended.
2. Form a loaf, then place in bottom of slow cooker.
3. Mix the sauce ingredients and pour into slow cooker. Cover, and cook for 6 hours at low temperature.

Nutrition information
Calories: 215
Fats: 8.89g
Carbohydrates: 21.74g
Proteins: 10.67g

Orange chicken

Ready in 1 h 30 minutes.
4 servings
11 Points

INGREDIENTS
- ¼ cup of all-purpose flour
- ¼ c. paprika
- 1/8 tsp. tea salt and pepper
- 2 pieces of chicken breast or (4 legs)
- 1 c. tablespoons butter
- 1 tsp. vegetable oil
- 4 carrots
- 1 onion cut into thin strips
- 2 tbsp. tablespoons brown sugar
- 2 cups of orange juice freshly squeezed
  - 1 cup sliced white mushrooms

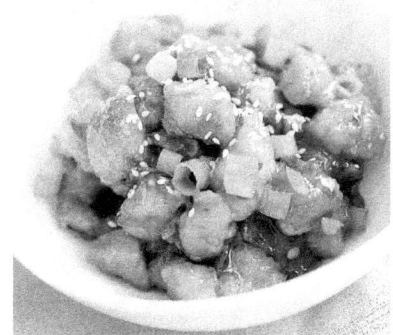

PREPARATION
1. Fry mushrooms in skillet and set aside to add to the very end. Mix flour, add salt, pepper, and coat the chicken.
2. Roast the chicken in hot oil and butter until golden brown, then remove from the pan and set aside.
3. In the same pan, fry all vegetables 4 to 5 minutes, stirring. Mix 3 tbsp. Soup of the previous flour mixture, brown sugar and stir vegetables for 1 minute. Pour the orange juice.
4. Return the chicken pieces to the pan, add the fried mushrooms, cover and cook for 1 hour or until chicken is tender.

Nutrition information
Calories: 380
Fats: 18g
Carbohydrates: 45g
Proteins: 14g

Steel-Cut Oats and Pumpkin

Prep time, 10 minutes. Cooking time, 6 hrs.
4 servings
5 Points

INREDIENTS
- 1 cup steel-cut oats
- 3 cups water
- 1 cup canned pumpkin puree
- Vanilla extract
- ½ cup honey and
- 2 tbsp. Tea Stevia

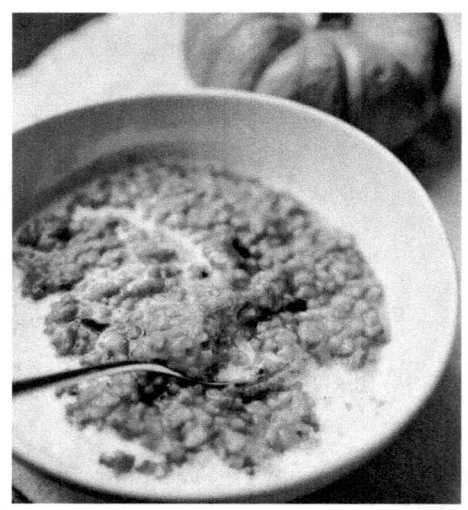

PREPARATION
1. Combine all ingredients in your Crock-Pot
2. Cook on low heat for 6 hours.

Nutrition information
Calories: 151.9
Fats: 1.5g
Carbohydrates: 34.5g
Proteins: 3.7g

Green Apple Jam, Quince and Cardamom

Prep time, 10 min. Cooking time, 8 hrs.
4 servings
2 Points

INGREDIENTS
- 32 oz. Granny Smith apple quince
- 1/3 oz. green cardamom
- ½ gallon of water
- 80 oz. sugar jam this jam is perfect with toast or waffles!

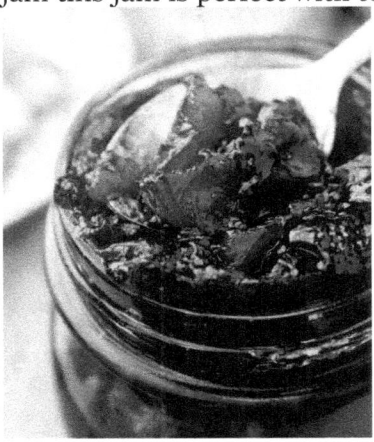

PREPARATION
1. Wash fruit and cut in half in one direction, then four in the other direction. Place the fruit in your Crock-Pot
2. Add water and cook at low heat for 8 hours. Add cardamom ½ hour before the end of cooking. Filter and drain the mixture in a clean, dry cloth to extract the most juice possible fruit pulps.
3. Transfer the extracted juice into a pan, followed by the sugar. Boil on your stove for ½ hour. Let cool overnight. The consistency of your jam will depend on the fruit quality and reduced time on the stove.

Nutrition information
Calories: 77.7
Fats: 0.1g
Carbohydrates: 20.4g
Proteins: 0.1g

Slow cooker toast

Prep time 5 min. Cooking time 8hrs.
5 servings.
5 Points

INGREDIENTS
- 1 loaf of sliced bread, no matter the kind
- 8-12 eggs
- 1 tsp. tablespoon vanilla extract
- 1 tsp. cinnamon
- 1 tsp. teaspoon brown sugar.

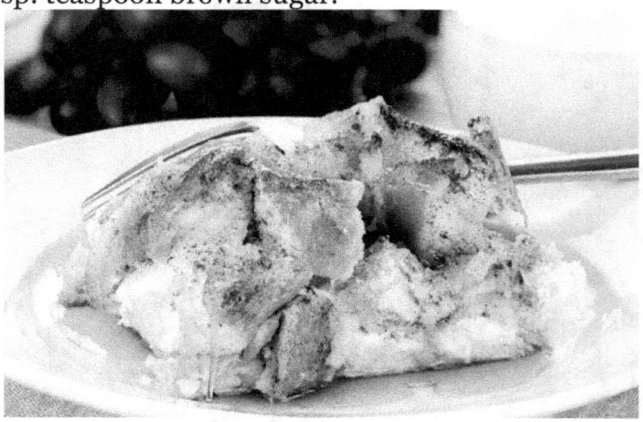

PREPARATION
- ✓ Grease the sides of the crock pot with butter.
- ✓ Place the loaf in the crock pot. Move the slices if the loaf is too big.
- ✓ In a bowl, combine eggs, vanilla, cinnamon and brown sugar.
- ✓ Pour mixture over bread, taking care to coat all pieces of bread
- ✓ Set the slow cooker on and cook for 6 to 8 hours.

Nutrition information
Calories: 163.1
Fats: 3.9g
Carbohydrates: 27.8g
Proteins: 6.4g

Sausage with tomatoes

Ready in 5h 30 min.
4 portions
6 Points

INGREDIENTS
- 1 1/2 lb. bacon sausage and beef
- 1 1/2 cup onions
- 3/4 cup chopped celery
- 1/3 cup flour
- 1 1/2 c. chili
- 1 1/2 c. sugar
- 1 1/2 c. Salt
- 1 can diced tomatoes
- 1 can tomato sauce
- 1 bay leaf

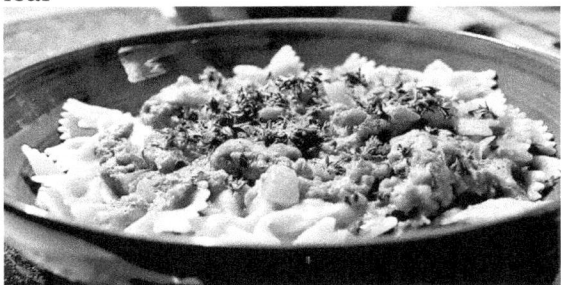

PREPARATION
1. In a skillet, brown the sausages slowly. Drain and place in slow cooker.
2. Fry the vegetables in the same pan used for sausages.
3. Add flour, chili powder, sugar and salt.
4. Sprinkle over fried vegetables.Add tomatoes and tomato sauce. Stir until the mixture is well blended and mixture becomes thicker.
5. Pour over sausage. Cook at low temperature of 5 to 7 hours.

Nutrition information
Calories: 222
Fats: 15g
Carbohydrates: 8g
Proteins: 14g

Spaghetti sauce with maple syrup

Ready in 5h 20 min.
10 portions
2 Points

INGREDIENTS
- 2 lb. lean ground beef
- 3 chopped carrots
- 3 stalks of celery, chopped
- 2 chopped green peppers
- 1 yellow pepper, chopped
- 1 large onion, finely chopped
- 1 small red onion, finely chopped
- 2 cans sliced mushrooms
- 1 clove garlic or 1/2 tsp.
- 1/4 cup barbecue sauce
- 1/2 cup chili sauce
- 3 c. tablespoons soy sauce
- 10 oz. diced tomatoes
- 10 oz. crushed tomatoes
- 9 oz. Hunt's tomato sauce
- 12 oz. tomato soup
- 1 box (small) tomato paste
- 1/2 cup maple syrup
- 3 pinches ground cloves
- 1/2 c. Tea Box crushed chili pepper
- 1/4 c. Tea marjoram
- 1 pinch cayenne pepper
- 3 drops tabasco
- 1/4 cup olive oil
- Salt and pepper

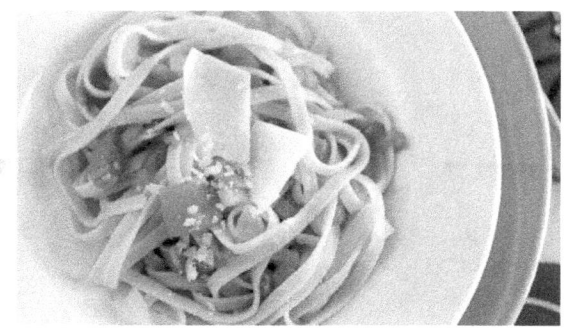

PREPARATION
1. Heat half the olive oil in a pan. Add ground beef, garlic, salt and pepper. Cover and cook over medium-low heat until cooked.
2. Meanwhile, put the vegetables in a pan with the remaining olive oil and sweat the vegetables over medium-low heat for 10 minutes (until the onion is transparent).
3. Set the slow cooker to low temperature. Add the tomato sauce, diced tomatoes, crushed tomatoes, BBQ sauce, soy sauce, chili sauce and tomato soup.
4. Add meat (with juices) and vegetables. Add spices, salt, pepper, Tabasco and tomato paste. Mix together and add maple syrup.
5. Cook for at least 5-6 hours in the slow cooker.

Nutrition information
Calories: 80
Fats: 3g
Carbohydrates: 11g
Proteins: 2g

Lemon Chicken

Ready in 8 h 20 min.
4 portions
6 Points

INGREDIENTS

- 2 cloves garlic, crushed
- 1 whole chicken
- 1 tablespoons dried oregano
- Pepper
- Salt
- 5 tablespoons water
- 2 tablespoons butter
- 4 tablespoon lemon juice
- 1 tablespoon of lemon zest

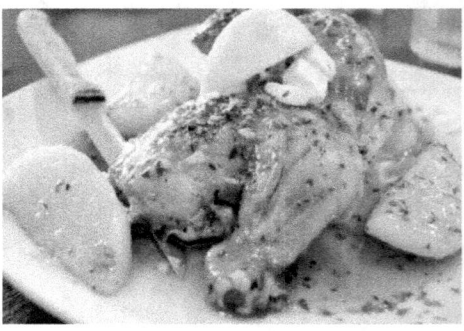

PREPARATION

1. Season chicken (inner part) with salt and pepper to taste.
2. Mix half of the oregano and garlic cloves. Rub the inside of the chicken with this mixture.
3. Melt butter in a skillet. Brown chicken on both sides. Then place it in the center of the slow cooker.
4. Sprinkle chicken with remaining oregano and the second garlic clove.
5. Add water to the pan to dissolve the chicken cooking residue. Then pour over chicken.
6. Cook the chicken at low temperature for 8 hours.
7. In the last hour of cooking, mix together the lemon juice and zest. Pour over chicken.
8. When the chicken is cooked, remove from the crock pot and serve.
9. Degrease the chicken and serve as a sauce.

Nutrition information
Calories: 226
Fats: 12g
Carbohydrates: 19g
Proteins: 11g

Prep time 10 min. Cooking time;6hrs.
6 servings
5 Points

INGREDIENTS
- 4 cups water
- 2 cups quinoa
- 2 cups blueberries
- 1/3 cup of chia seeds
- 1/3 cup honey

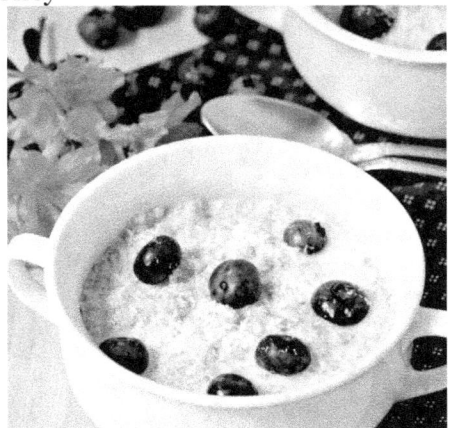

PREPARATION
1. Combine all ingredients in the bowl of slow cooker; cover and cook on low power (LOW) for 6-8 hours.

Nutrition information
Calories: 160
Fats: 2.5g
Carbohydrates: 33g
Proteins: 4g

Hot cider cranberries

Prep time 5 min. Cooking time; 20 min.
6 servings
2 Points

INGREDIENTS
- 2 liters of cranberry juice
- Zest of 2 oranges
- 14 cloves
- 1 1/2 cup dried cranberries
- 1 c. vanilla
- 1 1/3 cup honey
- 2 cinnamon sticks

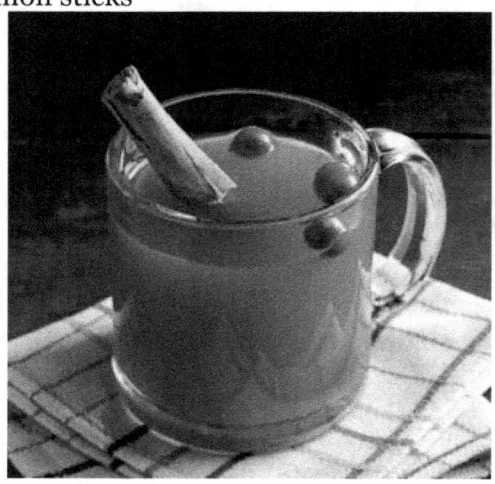

PREPARATION
1. Pour the cranberry juice in a slow cooker and set on high. Stir in the orange zest, nails, cranberries, vanilla, honey, and cinnamon sticks.
2. Cook, stirring occasionally, until the casserole is heated through, about 20 minutes.

Nutrition information
Calories: 79
Fats: 0.2g
Carbohydrates: 20g
Proteins: 0.1g

Prep time 10 min. Cooking time; 6 h.
20 servings.
3 Points

INGREDIENTS
- 2 liters of cranberry cocktail
- 3 cups orange juice
- 1/4 cup sugar
- 1/4 cup brown sugar
- 2 c. tablespoons fresh lemon juice
- a pinch of salt
- 2 inch cinnamon sticks

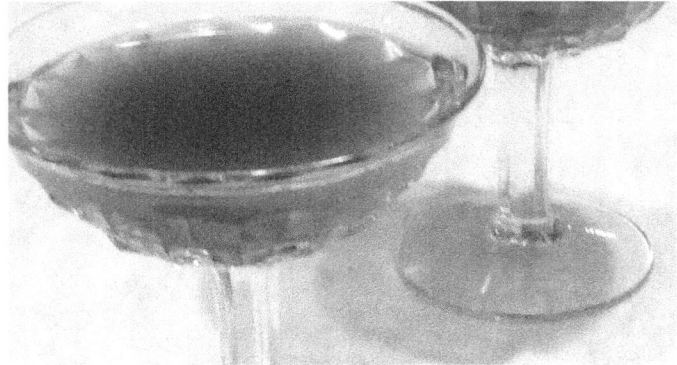

PREPARATION
1. Combine all ingredients in the bowl of the slow cooker and stir to dissolve the sugar and brown sugar.
2. Cook on high (HIGH) for 4-6 hours, then keep warm at low power for service.

Nutrition information
Calories: 124
Fats: 0.4g
Carbohydrates: 30.3g
Proteins: 0.6g

Chai tea

Prep time 15 min. Cooking time; 8 h.
16servings
7 Points

INGREDIENTS
- 3 1/2 liters of water
- 15 slices of fresh ginger, peeled
- 15 seeds of cardamom open and deseeded
- 25 whole cloves
- 3 cinnamon sticks
- 3 whole peppercorns
- 8 bags of black tea
- 1 can almond coconut milk

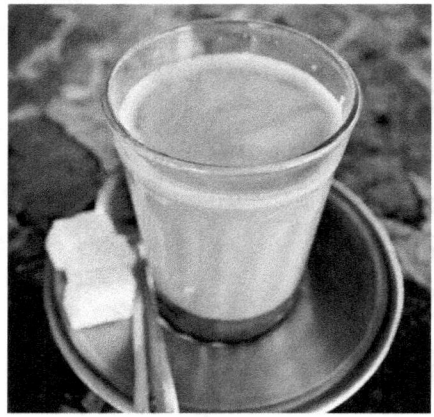

PREPARATION
1. Pour water into a slow cooker. Add ginger, cardamom pods, nails, cinnamon sticks and peppercorns. Microwave on high power and simmer for 8 hours.
2. Soak tea bags in the spicy water for 5 minutes. Place the tea strainer over a bowl. Add almond milk: Serve hot.

Nutrition information
Calories: 240
Fats: 4.5g
Carbohydrates: 45g
Proteins: 8g

Cocktail sausages

Prep time 10 min. Cooking time; 2 h.
6 servings
5 points

INGREDIENTS
- 2 ¼ cups BBQ sauce
- 1 cup packed brown sugar
- 1/2 cup ketchup
- 1 c. tablespoon Worcestershire sauce
- 1/3 cup chopped onion
- 4 packages (225 g each) cocktail sausages

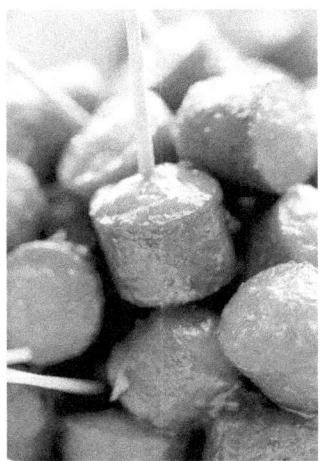

PREPARATION
1. Combine and mix all ingredients in the bowl of slow cooker. Cook on low for 2 hours.

Nutrition information
Calories: 206
Fats: 11g
Carbohydrates: 12g
Proteins: 12g

Slow Cooker Sausage Breakfast Casserole

Prep time 10 min. Cooking time; 8h.
6servings.
9 Points

INGREDIENTS

- 1 package frozen hash browns
- 1 package original hearty Sausage Crumbles
- 2 cup () of coconut milk
- 1/2 cup julienne cut, dried tomatoes packed in oil, drained
- 6 green onions, sliced
- 12 eggs
- 1/2 teaspoon salt
- 1/4 teaspoon ground black pepper

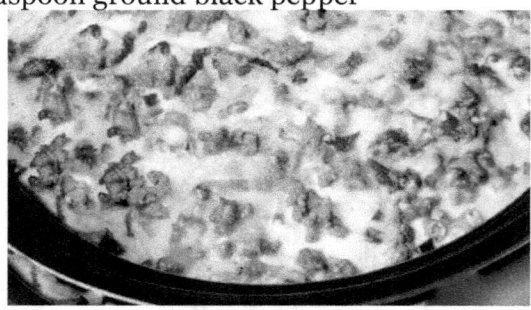

INSTRUCTIONS

1. Spray a slow cooker 6 quarter with cooking spray. Layer half of the potatoes in the bottom of the slow cooker.
2. Top the potatoes with half the sausage,, sundried tomatoes, and green onion. Repeat layering.
3. Beat eggs, coconut milk, salt and pepper in a large bowl with wire whisk until well blended.
4. Pour egg mixture evenly over the mixture of soil-sausage potatoes.
5. Cook on low for 8 hours or on high heat setting for four hours or until eggs are set.

Nutrition information
Calories: 334
Fats: 23g
Carbohydrates: 14g
Proteins: 17g

Potato gratin for breakfast

Prep time 10 min. Cooking time; 8h.
6 servings
6 Points

INGREDIENTS
- 2 cups water
- 5 potato wedges
- 0.25 cup all-purpose flour
- 1 teaspoon salt
- 0.13 teaspoon pepper
- 1.5 coconut milk

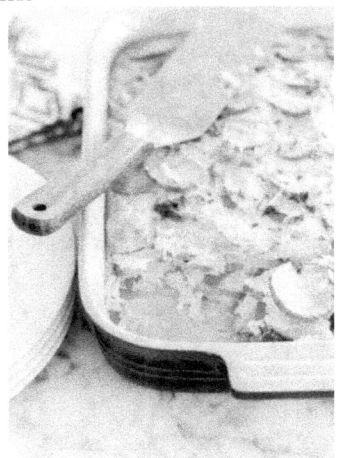

PREPARATION
1. Combine water and cream of tartar in a large bowl. Stir.
2. Add the potatoes. Stir well. Drain. Put the potatoes in a crock pot 5L.
3. Combine flour, salt and pepper.
4. Gradually stir in coconut milk, whisk until there are no more lumps. Heat, stirring, until mixture boils and thickens.
5. Cover. Cook on low for 6 to 8 hours.

Nutrition information
Calories: 240
Fats: 11g
Carbohydrates: 26g
Proteins: 7g

Slow Cooker Apple Cinnamon Oatmeal

Prep time 10 min. Cooking time; 8h.
2 servings.
4 Points

INGREDIENTS
- 1/2 cup oats
- 1/2 tsp. ground cinnamon
- 1/2 tsp. of vanilla extract
- A pinch of salt
- 2 cups water
- 1/2 small apple
- Unrefined sweetener

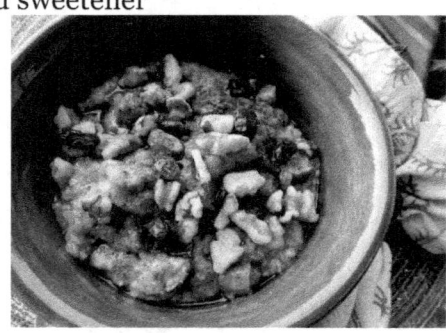

PREPARATION
1. In a small heat-proof bowl, stir together cinnamon, oats, vanilla, apples, and salt.
2. Pour two cups water over the oats.
3. Fill Slow Cooker about 1/2 of the way full with water.
4. Add the heatproof bowl containing oat mixture to the Slow Cooker.
5. Cook on low heat for 7-8 hours overnight. Remove bowl from Slow Cooker.
6. Add sweetener of your choice.

Nutrition information
Calories: 130
Fats: 1.5g
Carbohydrates: 27g
Proteins: 3g

Prep time 15 min. Cooking time; 8h.
6 servings
6 Points

INGREDIENTS
- 3 cups vegetable stock
- 14 oz. diced tomatoes
- 14 oz. coconut milk
- 1 cup dry green lentils
- 1/2 cup dry red lentils
- 2 cups butternut squash, peeled, seeded and diced
- 1 onion, chopped
- 1 jalapeno pepper
- 1 tsp. Chili powder
- 1/4 tsp. Ground cumin
- 1/4 tsp. Ground coriander
- 1/4 tsp. Ground turmeric
- Salt and pepper

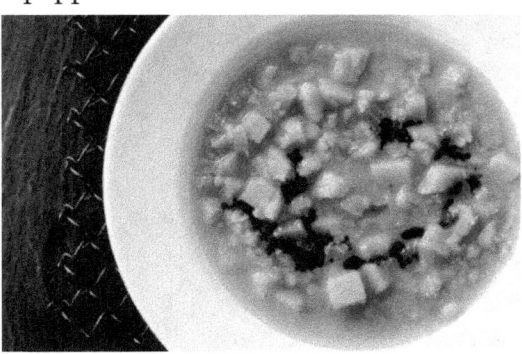

PREPARATION
- ✓ In slow cooker, combine all ingredients.
- ✓ Add Salt and pepper. Cover and cook at low temperature for 6 hours. We can maintain stove (Warm) to 8 hours.
- ✓ Serve with bread.

Nutrition information
Calories: 230
Fats: 6g
Carbohydrates: 27.3g
Proteins: 15.4g

Apple quinoa porridge

Prep time 5 min. Cooking time; 2h.
3 servings
6 Points

INGREDIENTS

- 1 cup red quinoa, rinsed and drained
- 1 apple, peeled
- 1/2 c. teaspoon salt
- 1 c. of cinnamon
- 2 c. tablespoons maple syrup
- 1/3 cup slivered almonds
- 1 ½ cups almond milk

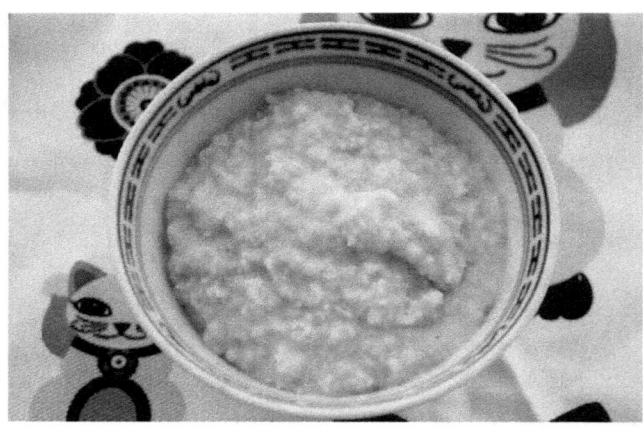

PREPARATION

1. Combine the quinoa and water in a slow cooker. Bring to boil, reduce heat to medium, cover and simmer until the quinoa is tender, 45 minutes.
2. Add the apple and sprinkle with salt, cinnamon and maple syrup. Add almonds; cook until apples soften, 30 minutes. Add the almond milk and cream; heat through. Add cooked quinoa and cook for 30 minutes.
3. Warm up a few minutes before serving.

Nutrition information
Calories: 220
Fats: 3g
Carbohydrates: 39g
Proteins: 10g

Breakfast oats

Prep time 5 min. Cooking time; 9h.
3 servings.
4 Points

INGREDIENTS
- 2 cups of oatmeal
- 2 apples
- 1 tsp. cinnamon
- 4 cups of water

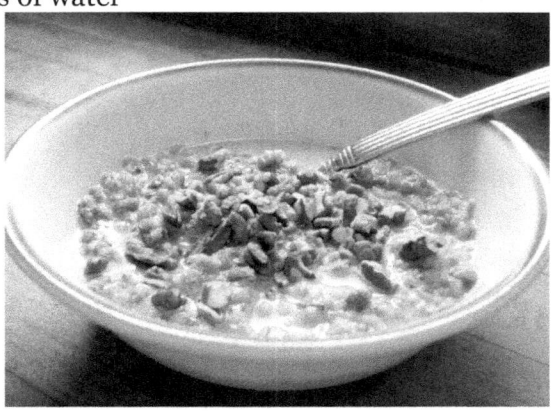

PREPARATION
1. Pour all ingredients in a slow cooker. Do NOT stir.
2. Cook overnight for 8 – 9 hours on low.

Nutrition information
Calories: 150
Fats: 2.5g
Carbohydrates: 27g
Proteins: 5g

Ranchers roast beef

Ready after 9 hours
4 servings
5 Points

INGREDIENTS
- ¼ pepperoncini juice
- ½ teaspoon of kosher salt
- 1 packet ranch dressing mix
- 2 Cups of beef broth
- 2 tablespoon butter
- ½ sliced pepperoncini
- 1 tablespoon corn starch
- 2 tablespoon canola oil
- ½ Cup sour cream
- 2-3 lb. beef chuck roast

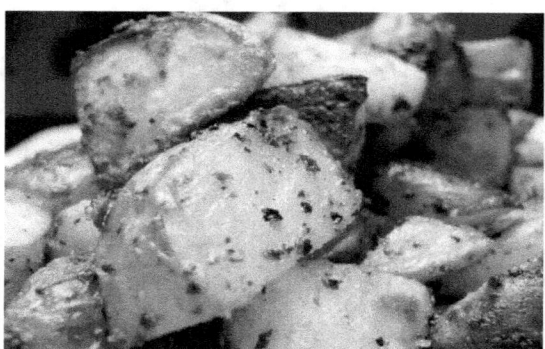

PREPARATION
1. Over medium heat, heat canola oil. Use pepper and salt to season the roast and cook in hot oil up to the point it is golden brown.
2. Put the roast into a crock pot and add the dressing mixture as you sprinkle (pepperoncini juice, butter and pepperoncini)
3. Adjust to low heat and cook on the crock pot for 8 hours. Get the meat of the pot and pour the juices into a saucepan. Get rid of the excess fat by skimming.
4. To the juices, add beef broth and heat to boil.
5. Make a mixture of ¼ cup of water, and 1 tablespoon cornstarch and add it to the mixture of beef broth. Heat as

you stir until it thickens. Stop heating then add ½ cup of sour cream as you stir to make it thicker. Serve over meat that is already cooked.

Nutrition information
Calories: 195
Fats: 12g
Carbohydrates: 14g
Proteins: 5g

BBQ beef sandwich

Ready after 8 hours 30 minutes
4 servings
8 Points

INREDIENTS
- 2 tablespoons Dijon mustard
- 1 cups ketchup
- 1/4 cup barbecue sauce
- 1/2 teaspoon of salt
- 1 teaspoon of Liquid Smoke
- 1/4 teaspoon garlic powder
- 2 tablespoons Worcestershire sauce
- 1/4 teaspoon pepper
- 12 sandwich buns, split
- 1/4 cup packed brown sugar
- Sliced onions and pickled jalapenos (not a must)
- 1 boneless beef chuck roast

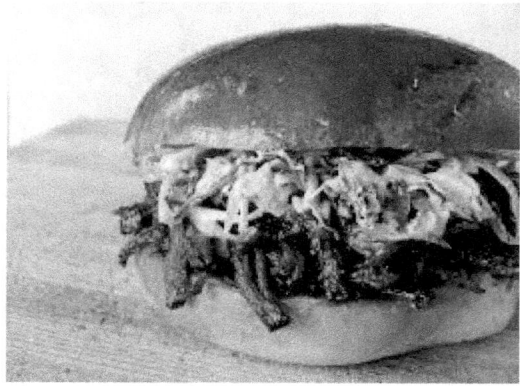

PREPARATION
1. Take the roast and cutting it into halves, place it in your slow cooker. Make a brown sugar mixture Worcestershire sauce, ketchup, liquid smoke, seasonings and mustard in a small bowl.
1. Add the mixture to the beef. Cook for about eight hours while covering. Allow the meat to cool as you remove the fat from the liquid by skimming.
2. Use two forks to shred the beef then put it in the slow cooker. Cook for fifteen minutes while covered. Place half a cup on each bun using a slotted spoon. You could serve with jalapenos or onions.

Nutrition information
Calories: 325
Fats: 15g
Carbohydrates: 16g
Proteins: 30g

CONCLUSION

With the plump chaps who lament about how they "eat all day and still can't lose weight," it's not surprising for them to get a small slice of ordinary pie when dining. You can unquestionably loose pounds in a healthy way. I'm animated that you are looking for the right way to lose weight without restricting yourself to some foods.Weight watchers diet has been mentioned as the latest trend to achieve all your fitness goals. Don't be left behind! Enjoy these amazing meal ideas as they will see you hit your fitness target.

Thank you for downloading this book. Kindly leave a comment on the feedback section.

Before You Go

If you liked this book you may like these other books from **Henry White**

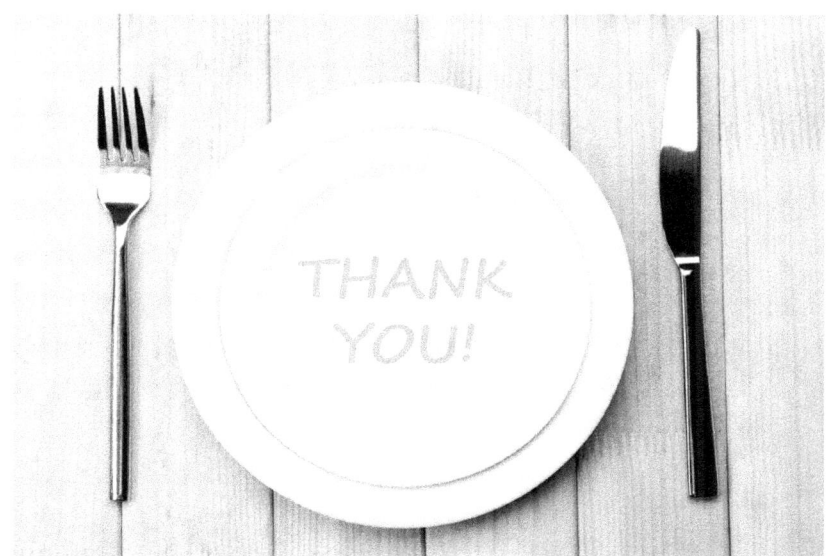

Did you enjoy this book?

I want to thank you for purchasing and reading this book. I really hope you got a lot out of it.

Can I ask a quick favor through?

If you enjoyed this book I would really appreciate ii if you could leave me an honest review on Amazon.